Pathophysiology of **<u>Heart Disease</u>**
(made easy)

Straight forward guide to learn for Medical Students, Nurses, Physicians, and other Healthcare Professionals (all you must know)

Louis M. Lilly

Table of Contents

- CHAPTER ONE 3
  - Introduction 3
- CHAPTER TWO 8
  - Risk Factors for Heart Disease 8
  - Atherosclerosis: The Underlying Process 16
- CHAPTER THREE 20
  - Chronic Inflammation 20
  - Coronary Artery Disease (CAD) 25
- CHAPTER FOUR 34
  - Heart Failure 34
  - Other Heart Conditions 44
- CHAPTER FIVE 51
  - Congenital Heart Defect Types 51

Cellular and Molecular Mechanisms of Heart Disease 54

CHAPTER SIX 57

Defenses Against Antioxidants 57

THE END 66

CHAPTER ONE
Introduction
Heart Disease Definition

Heart disease, also referred to as cardiovascular disease (CVD), is a broad term for a number of disorders affecting the heart and blood arteries. Heart failure, arrhythmias, coronary artery disease, and congenital heart abnormalities are among these ailments. The most prevalent kind, coronary artery disease, is characterized by the constriction or obstruction of the coronary arteries, typically as a result of atherosclerosis. Heart attacks, strokes, and even death are among the serious health issues that can result from heart disease. It continues to be one of the main causes of illness and death globally, thus a thorough understanding of its many manifestations and underlying mechanisms is necessary.

Importance of Understanding Pathophysiology

It is essential to comprehend the pathophysiology of cardiac disease for a number of reasons:

Diagnosis and Treatment: Accurate diagnosis of various forms of heart disease and customization of treatment regimens to target individual pathologies are made possible by healthcare professionals' understanding of the underlying mechanisms. This can guarantee prompt and suitable interventions, which can enhance patient outcomes.

Prevention: Researchers and physicians can find risk factors and early illness signs by studying the pathophysiology of heart disease. With the goal of lowering the incidence of heart disease, preventative measures such as medicine, lifestyle changes, and public health campaigns can be developed thanks to this knowledge.

Research and Innovation: Scientific research and innovation are driven by insights into the pathophysiology of cardiac disease. This may result in the identification of fresh therapeutic targets, the advancement of diagnostic technologies, and the development of cutting-edge therapies. To fight the ever-evolving issues connected with heart disease, research must continue.

Education and Awareness: Raising knowledge about the mechanisms underlying heart disease among the general public and medical professionals helps to promote awareness and understanding. Improved health literacy may result from this, motivating people to adopt healthier habits and seek medical assistance when needed.

To sum up, enhancing diagnosis, treatment, prevention, and research endeavors requires a solid grasp of the pathophysiology of heart disease. It is essential for lessening the effects of this common and frequently fatal group of illnesses.

CHAPTER TWO
Risk Factors for Heart Disease

Changeable Risk Elements

Heart disease risk factors that can be altered by dietary adjustments or therapeutic interventions are known as modifiable risk factors. By taking care of these issues, heart disease risk might be considerably decreased.

Cholesterol and Diet

Poor Diet: Eating a diet heavy in cholesterol, saturated and trans fats, sugar, and salt raises the risk of heart disease. These food items may contribute to the fatty deposit accumulation in the arteries that is known as atherosclerosis.

High concentrations of low-density lipoprotein (LDL) cholesterol, which is commonly known as "bad" cholesterol, have been linked to the development of plaque in the arteries. On the other hand, elevated levels of "good" cholesterol, or high-density lipoprotein (HDL), aid in the elimination of cholesterol from the blood.

Blood Pressure

High blood pressure, or hypertension, is a major cause of heart disease risk. It makes the heart work harder to pump blood, which over time may cause the heart muscle to thicken and the blood vessels to deteriorate.

Diabetes

Heart disease is more common in those who have diabetes. Elevated blood sugar levels have the potential to harm heart-controlling neurons and blood arteries. Cardiovascular problems are substantially more likely in people with diabetes, including Type 1 and Type 2.

Being overweight

Diabetes, high blood pressure, and high cholesterol are a few heart disease risk factors that are linked to obesity. Overweight is associated with a higher risk of heart disease, especially around the belly.

Consuming tobacco

One of the main risk factors for heart disease is smoking. Tobacco smoke contains chemicals that harm the heart and blood arteries, causing atherosclerosis. Additionally, smoking lowers blood oxygen levels, which raises heart rate and blood pressure.

Absence of Exercise

Heart disease is significantly increased by physical inactivity.

Frequent exercise improves cardiovascular health overall, decreases blood pressure, lowers cholesterol, and helps people maintain a healthy weight.

Non-Adaptable Risk Elements

Risk variables that are immutable are those that people are powerless to alter. Understanding these variables is crucial for identifying those who are more vulnerable and putting the right preventative measures in place.

Age

As people age, their risk of heart disease rises. People who are older may be more susceptible to cardiovascular diseases due to changes in their heart and blood vessels. Women over 55 and males over 45 are more vulnerable.

Molecular Biology

The risk of heart disease can be influenced by genetic factors. Blood pressure, atherosclerosis susceptibility, and cholesterol levels can all be impacted by certain genetic variants. Familial hypercholesterolemia is one hereditary illness that dramatically raises the risk of heart disease.

Ancestral History

A family history of heart disease is a strong risk factor. People who have close family members (parents, siblings) who experienced early-onset heart disease (before the age of 55 for men and before the age of 65 for women) are more vulnerable. This raises the possibility of a genetic susceptibility and common lifestyle elements.

It is imperative to comprehend and effectively manage modifiable as well as non-modifiable risk variables in order to prevent heart disease and enhance cardiovascular health. People can greatly lower their risk and improve their general health by adopting new lifestyle habits, getting frequent checkups, and using medical interventions.

Atherosclerosis: The Underlying Process

The buildup of plaque inside the artery walls is the hallmark of the complicated and progressive disease known as atherosclerosis. The arteries constrict and stiffen as a result of this process, which can seriously impair blood flow and cause a number of cardiovascular problems.

Development of a Plaque

Endothelial Damage

Damage to the endothelium, the inner lining of the arteries, is the first step toward atherosclerosis. Factors including smoking, diabetes, high blood pressure, excessive cholesterol, and inflammation can all contribute to this damage. Endothelial damage draws inflammatory cells and increases the permeability of arterial walls to lipoproteins.

Buildup of Lipoproteins

Low-density lipoprotein (LDL) cholesterol builds up in the artery wall after penetrating the injured endothelium. After entering the body, LDL cholesterol experiences oxidative alteration, transforming into highly atherogenic oxidized LDL (ox-LDL) that can promote atherosclerosis.

inflammatory reaction

When ox-LDL is present, an inflammatory reaction is triggered. White blood cells called monocytes move to the area of damage and undergo macrophage differentiation there. These macrophages become foam cells when they absorb ox-LDL. The first noticeable sign of atherosclerosis is a fatty streak, which is created when foam cells build up.

Formation of Plaques

Smooth muscle cells move and multiply over time from the arterial media (middle layer) to the intima (inner layer). These cells help to establish a fibrous cap over the fatty stripe by producing extracellular matrix components including collagen and elastin. A developed atherosclerotic plaque is composed of smooth muscle cells, foam cells, and extracellular matrix.

The Function of Inflammation

From the earliest phases of atherosclerosis to its advancement and final plaque rupture, inflammation is a key factor in all of these processes. Important elements consist of:

CHAPTER THREE
Chronic Inflammation

The cycle of damage and repair is sustained by the persistent inflammatory response, which also encourages more immune cell recruitment and endothelial dysfunction. The plaque is driven by persistent inflammation.

Release of Cytokine

Cytokines and chemokines are released by inflammatory cells; these signaling molecules draw additional immune cells to the site of injury and promote the growth of smooth muscle cells. Leukocyte adhesion and migration are aided by these cytokines, which also cause endothelial cells to produce adhesion molecules.

MMPs, or matrix metalloproteinases

MMPs are enzymes produced by inflammatory cells that break down the extracellular matrix. This deterioration may weaken the fibrous cap and increase the likelihood of a rupture.

The Effects of Plaque Deposition

Vascular Constriction

Blood flow is decreased as the plaque thickens and narrows the artery lumen. Insufficient blood flow, or ischemia, may result in the tissues that are supplied by the impacted artery. This may result in angina (chest pain) in coronary arteries.

Breakage of the Plaque

The underlying thrombogenic material in the plaque may become visible to the bloodstream when the fibrous cap covering it ruptures. At the site of rupture, this exposure causes a blood clot, or thrombus, to form, which can quickly clog the artery.

Acute Heart Conditions

Acute coronary syndromes, such as myocardial infarction, can occur when a thrombus substantially or totally obstructs a coronary artery (heart attack). Stroke can result from cerebral artery plaque rupture and the thrombus that forms after it.

The Ischemic Peripheral Arteries

Peripheral artery disease (PAD), which can cause pain, ulceration, and even gangrene, is a result of atherosclerosis in the arteries feeding the limbs.

To summarize, endothelial damage, lipid buildup, and

persistent inflammation are the three main factors that drive the dynamic process of atherosclerosis. Plaque accumulation can lead to artery constriction, plaque rupture, and thrombus formation, all of which significantly increase the risk of cardiovascular events like heart attacks and strokes. It is essential to comprehend this process in order to create prevention and treatment plans for atherosclerosis.

Coronary Artery Disease (CAD)

A form of cardiovascular disease called coronary artery disease (CAD) mostly affects the coronary arteries, which provide blood to the heart muscle (myocardium). Atherosclerosis, a disorder marked by the accumulation of plaque in the arterial walls, is the main cause of coronary artery disease (CAD).

The Impact of Atherosclerosis on Coronary Arteries

The same basic mechanisms that cause atherosclerosis in other arteries also affect the coronary arteries, but because the heart is constantly pumping blood and oxygen, the effects of atherosclerosis are especially severe.

Formation of Plaques

First, there is injury to the endothelial cells that line the coronary arteries, which causes LDL cholesterol to build up and fatty streaks to form.

Immune cells are drawn to inflammatory responses and absorb oxidized low-density lipoprotein (LDL), converting into foam cells and creating plaque.

Growth of Plaques and Arterial Narrowing

As plaques enlarge and extend into the artery lumen, the arteries become narrower and the myocardium's blood supply is restricted. The medical term for this ailment is coronary artery stenosis.

The degree of constriction can range from modest to severe, which can have an impact on the heart's capacity to take in enough oxygen, particularly when there is a surge in demand, like during stressful or physically demanding moments.

Closure of the Plaque and Thrombosis

A thrombus, or blood clot, is formed when a plaque bursts, exposing its contents to the bloodstream. This may cause the coronary artery to become acutely blocked, severely reducing blood flow.

Pectorile Angina

Chest pain or discomfort, generally known as angina pectoris or angina, is caused by a deficiency of oxygen-rich blood flow to the myocardium.

Consistent Angina

Features: Rest or nitroglycerin cure stable angina, which happens predictably in response to physical exertion or mental stress.

Mechanism: Usually brought on by a stable, fixed plaque that narrows the coronary arteries, it restricts blood flow while the heart is working harder.

Unsteady Angina

Features: Unstable angina is erratic, can strike during rest or with little effort, and is not easily eased by medication or sleep. It could be a warning sign of a heart attack.

Mechanism: It is caused by a large but incomplete restriction of blood flow resulting from a partly occlusive thrombus caused by plaque rupture or erosion.

cardiac arrest, or myocardial infarction

Heart attacks, often referred to as myocardial infarctions (MI), happen when blood flow is cut off to a portion of the heart muscle for a lengthy length of time, leading to necrosis or tissue destruction.

MI Mechanism

Thrombosis and Plaque Rupture: The most frequent cause of MI is the rupture of an atherosclerotic plaque in a coronary artery, which is followed by the development of a thrombus that blocks the artery entirely.

Ischemia and Infarction: An extended period of blood supply deprivation causes myocardial cells to die (infarction). The length of the blockage, the size, and the placement of the blocked artery all affect how much harm is done.

MI symptoms

Severe, ongoing chest pain or discomfort that is frequently described as a tightness, pressure, or squeezing sensation. The jaw, neck, back, arms, or shoulders may all experience radiating pain.

Additional symptoms include anxiety, sweating, nausea, vomiting, dizziness, and shortness of breath. Atypical symptoms in women can include weariness, dizziness, and stomach pain.

MI Complications

Heart Failure: Impairments to the heart muscle's capacity to pump blood efficiently can result in heart failure.

Arrhythmias: Abnormal heart rhythms can be potentially fatal when there is a disruption in the heart's electrical activity.

Cardiogenic Shock: Serious cardiac damage can result in a

significant drop in blood flow, which can cause organ failure and necessitate immediate medical attention.

In conclusion, coronary artery disease has a major negative impact on heart health due to the processes of atherosclerosis, which result in disorders like myocardial infarction and angina pectoris. In order to lower the risk of major cardiovascular events, it is imperative to comprehend these pathways in order to prevent, diagnose, and treat CAD.

CHAPTER FOUR
Heart Failure

A chronic illness known as heart failure occurs when the heart cannot pump enough blood to meet the body's demands. It can be caused by a number of cardiac conditions, such as cardiomyopathies, hypertension, and coronary artery disease. The kind of malfunction and the particular stage of the cardiac cycle that is compromised are the two main factors used to categorize heart failure.

Dysfunction, Systolic vs. Diastolic

Heart Failure with Reduced Ejection Fraction, or HFrEF, is known as systolic dysfunction.

Definition: Systolic dysfunction is the loss of the heart muscle's capacity to contract powerfully enough to pump enough blood during the contraction phase, or systole.

Mechanism: A decreased ejection fraction (EF), or the proportion of blood that the heart expels with each contraction, is the hallmark of this illness. Systolic dysfunction is usually indicated by an EF of less than 40%.

Causes: Dilated cardiomyopathy, persistent hypertension, and ischemic heart disease (such as myocardial infarction) are common causes.

Heart Failure with Preserved Ejection Fraction, or HFpEF, is known as diastolic dysfunction.

Definition: Diastolic dysfunction is the insufficient filling of the ventricles caused by stiff heart muscle that is unable to relax during diastole, the relaxation phase.

Mechanism: Impaired ventricular relaxation and elevated filling pressures prevent the heart from filling with adequate blood, even in cases when the ejection fraction is normal or almost normal (often above 50%).

Causes: Aging-related alterations in the cardiac muscle, hypertrophic cardiomyopathy, and persistent hypertension are common causes.

Remodeling of the Heart

The term "myocardial remodeling" describes anatomical and functional alterations in the heart brought on by long-term stress or cardiac damage. These alterations may at first be adaptive, but they frequently turn maladaptive and accelerate the development of heart failure.

Unhealthy Remodeling

Hypertrophy: As in the cases of aortic stenosis and hypertension, the heart's myocytes (or heart muscle cells) grow to make up for an increased workload. This results in hypertrophy, or thickening of the heart walls, which can affect diastolic and systolic function.

Fibrosis: When fibrous tissue accumulates in the heart muscle, it loses some of its elasticity and contractility, which exacerbates diastolic dysfunction and raises the possibility of arrhythmias.

Dilation: The heart chambers dilate in reaction to a persistent volume excess, such as that which occurs in dilated cardiomyopathy or mitral regurgitation. This keeps the cardiac output stable at first, but when the heart's capacity to pump becomes less, it finally causes systolic dysfunction.

Modifications in Molecular Structure

Neurohormonal Activation: Renin-angiotensin-aldosterone system (RAAS) and sympathetic nervous system activation are brought on by chronic heart failure and can worsen remodeling. Angiotensin II and aldosterone excesses stimulate cardiac cell hypertrophy, fibrosis, and apoptosis (death of the cell).

Heart Failure's Clinical Presentation

Heart failure can manifest clinically in a variety of ways, but typical indications and symptoms include:

Symptoms

Dyspnea: Breathlessness, particularly when exerting oneself (exertional dyspnea) or when in a prone position (orthopnea). An abrupt and severe dyspnea occurs at night and is known as paroxysmal nocturnal dyspnea (PND).

Fatigue and Weakness: As a result of decreased blood supply to muscles and tissues as well as decreased cardiac output.

Edema: Fluid retention-related swelling in the legs, ankles, and feet (peripheral edema). Ascites, or a buildup of fluid in the belly, and pleural effusion, or fluid surrounding the lungs, can happen in extreme situations.

Cough and Wheezing: Fluid buildup in the lungs, also known

as pulmonary congestion, can be the cause of a persistent cough or wheezing that is frequently worse at night.

Indications

Increased central venous pressure is indicated by elevated pressure in the jugular veins, which is known as jugular vein distention (JVD).

Rales or Crackles: Abnormal breath sounds detected during auscultation that suggest the presence of fluid in the lungs' alveoli.

S3 Heart Sound: Often linked to heart failure, this additional heart sound, often known as the third heart sound, is audible during fast ventricular filling.

Hepatomegaly and Hepatojugular Reflux: Right-sided heart failure indicated by an enlarged liver and a positive hepatojugular reflux test.

Effective diagnosis and treatment of heart failure depend on an understanding of its causes and clinical manifestations. The course of treatment usually entails addressing the underlying reasons, changing one's lifestyle, taking medications to manage symptoms and limit the disease's progression, and occasionally undergoing surgery.

Other Heart Conditions
Arrhythmias: irregular heartbeats

Abnormal cardiac rhythms are caused by diseases of the heart's electrical system, known as arrhythmias. They can be categorized according to the aberrant rhythm's source (ventricular or atrial) or heart rate (tachyarrhythmias and bradyarrhythmias), and they can range in severity from benign to life-threatening.

Synchronized heartbeats

The most frequent kind of arrhythmia, atrial fibrillation (AFib), is characterized by the atria pounding rapidly and irregularly. It raises the risk of heart failure and stroke.

SVT, or supraventricular tachycardia, is a fast heartbeat that starts above the ventricles and frequently results in palpitations, lightheadedness, and chest pain.

Ventricular tachycardia (VT) is a fast heartbeat that starts in the ventricles. It can be fatal and lead to ventricular fibrillation (VFib), which is a condition that needs to be treated right away.

Bradyarrhythmias

A slow heartbeat brought on by the sinoatrial (SA) node

discharging more slowly than usual is known as sinus bradycardia. In athletes, it can be normal, but if it's accompanied by other symptoms like weariness or dizziness, it might be a sign of trouble.

Heart Block: An electrical impulse that delays or stops entirely as it passes through the heart's conduction pathway. Heart blocks come in three different types: first-degree, second-degree (Mobitz types I and II), and third-degree (complete).

Presenting Clinically with Arrhythmias

Palpitations, lightheadedness, vertigo, syncope, chest discomfort, and dyspnea are among the symptoms.

Holter monitoring, electrocardiograms (ECGs), and event recorders are used in the diagnosis. Electrophysiological investigations could be carried out for a more thorough evaluation.

Heart Valve Disease

The mitral, aortic, tricuspid, or pulmonary valves are the four heart valves that can sustain injury or malfunction in patients with valvular heart disease. This may lead to regurgitation, or valve leakage, or stenosis, or narrowing of the valve.

Mitral Valve Disorder

Mitral Stenosis: Reduced blood flow from the left atrium to the left ventricle due to narrowing of the mitral valve, typically brought on by rheumatic fever.

Mitral regurgitation: During systole, blood flows backward into the left atrium due to a malfunctioning mitral valve.

Disease of the Aortic Valve

Aortic Stenosis: Narrowing of the aortic valve that obstructs blood flow from the left ventricle to the aorta, frequently brought on by calcification associated with aging.

Aortic regurgitation occurs when the aortic valve malfunctions, causing blood to return to the left ventricle during diastole.

Additional Valvular Conditions

Less frequently occurring but potentially causing stenosis or regurgitation, which impairs blood flow to the right side of the heart, are tricuspid and pulmonary valve diseases.

The clinical manifestation of heart valve disease

Symptoms may include syncope, palpitations, exhaustion, dyspnea, and dyspnea. Heart failure may result from severe cases.

The main diagnostic method is the echocardiogram. Additional information can be obtained via cardiac catheterization, MRI, and CT scans.

Birth Heart Problems

Congenital heart defects (CHDs) are variations in the structure of the heart that exist from birth. They can be as simple as having no symptoms or as complex as having severe, potentially fatal symptoms.

CHAPTER FIVE
Congenital Heart Defect Types

Septal Defects: Hole in the septum of the heart. Common kinds of atrial and ventricular septal defects (ASD and VSD, respectively) cause irregular blood flow between the chambers.

Patent Ductus Arteriosus (PDA): This condition is caused by an irregular blood flow between the aorta and the pulmonary artery. The ductus arteriosus is a conduit that bypasses fetal lung circulation. It fails to shut after birth.

Tetralogy of Fallot: Right ventricular hypertrophy, pulmonary stenosis, an overriding aorta, and ventriculosnic dilation. It makes blood that is deficient in oxygen leave the heart and flow throughout the body.

Transposition of the Great Arteries (TGA): When the aorta and pulmonary arteries are positioned incorrectly, blood that is both deoxygenated and oxygenated cannot circulate properly.

Congenital Heart Defects' Clinical Presentation

Symptoms include heart murmurs, fast breathing, poor feeding, cyanosis (a bluish tinge to the skin), and failure to thrive.

The diagnosis was made using cardiac catheterization, MRI, chest X-ray, echocardiography, and prenatal ultrasound.

In order to enhance patient outcomes and quality of life, understanding and managing these diverse cardiac problems requires a multidisciplinary strategy that includes lifestyle modifications, medicines, surgical procedures, and routine monitoring.

Cellular and Molecular Mechanisms of Heart Disease

Oxidative Stress's Function

One important factor in the pathophysiology of cardiac disease is oxidative stress. It happens when the body's capacity to eliminate these reactive intermediates or heal the harm they cause is out of balance with the generation of reactive oxygen species (ROS).

ROS Sources in the Heart

The main source of ROS in cardiomyocytes is mitochondria. Superoxide anions may develop as a result of electron leakage during oxidative phosphorylation.

NADPH Oxidases: Enzymes that generate ROS during typical signaling pathways within cells.

Xanthine Oxidase: A purine metabolism-related enzyme that produces reactive oxygen species.

Under some pathological situations, Uncoupled Nitric Oxide Synthase (NOS) produces superoxide instead of nitric oxide.

ROS effects

Lipid Peroxidation: ROS have the ability to cause lipid peroxidation, which damages cellular membranes by causing a loss of membrane integrity and cellular malfunction.

Protein Oxidation: Reactive oxygen species (ROS) can change the structure and function of amino acids in proteins, hence compromising the structural integrity of proteins and the activity of enzymes.

DNA Damage: ROS have the ability to break DNA strands and change bases, which can result in mutations and apoptosis.

CHAPTER SIX
Defenses Against Antioxidants

Enzymatic antioxidants: Catalase, glutathione peroxidase, and superoxide dismutase (SOD) are essential for detoxifying reactive oxygen species (ROS).

Non-enzymatic Antioxidants: Coenzyme Q10, glutathione, and vitamins C and E assist in preventing ROS and safeguarding cellular constituents.

Effects on the Function of Cardiomyocytes

Cardiomyocyte function is negatively impacted by oxidative stress via multiple mechanisms:

Reduced Flexibility

ROS have the ability to alter proteins that play a role in excitation-contraction coupling, including calcium channels and ryanodine receptors. This can cause abnormalities in calcium homeostasis and reduced contractility.

Necrosis and Apoptosis

Cardiomyocytes may undergo necrosis, or uncontrollably dying cells, or planned cell death, as a result of excessive oxidative stress.

Caspases are activated, cytochrome c is released, and mitochondrial damage are the processes that mediate apoptosis.

dysfunction of the mitochondria

ROS have the ability to harm proteins and DNA in the mitochondria, which impairs ATP synthesis and increases ROS production in turn, resulting in a vicious cycle of oxidative stress and mitochondrial malfunction.

Inflammatory response

Tissue damage can be exacerbated by ROS-induced activation of inflammatory signaling pathways, which results in the generation of pro-inflammatory cytokines and the infiltration of immune cells.

The Signaling Channels Involved

Numerous signaling pathways are essential in the development of heart disease and are involved in the physiological response to oxidative stress.

The pathway of Nuclear Factor Kappa B (NF-κB)

NF-κB is a transcription factor that controls the expression of genes related to inflammation, immunological response, and cell survival. ROS can activate this transcription factor.

Effect: Long-term NF-κB activation causes persistent inflammation, which advances atherosclerosis, myocardial infarction, and heart failure.

The pathway of Mitogen-Activated Protein Kinase (MAPK)

Extracellular signal-regulated kinases (ERK), c-Jun N-terminal kinases (JNK), and p38 MAPK are among the components.

Function: These kinases mediate responses such cell proliferation, differentiation, death, and inflammation. They are activated by oxidative stress.

Impact: Pathological remodeling and cardiomyocyte death may result from persistent stimulation.

The PI3K/Akt Pathway

Function: The proliferation and survival of cells are impacted by this pathway. ROS have the ability to alter this route, which, depending on the situation, may have beneficial or negative consequences.

Impact: PI3K/Akt activation can shield cells from oxidative damage and increase cell survival. Chronic stimulation, however, might be a factor in pathological hypertrophy.

The pathway of AMP-Activated Protein Kinase (AMPK)

Activation: Elevated AMP/ATP ratios, which are frequently the consequence of oxidative stress, activate AMPK.

Function: By increasing mitochondrial biogenesis, fatty acid oxidation, and glucose absorption, AMPK supports energy homeostasis.

Impact: AMPK activation has preventive effects against heart disease by reducing oxidative stress and enhancing cellular energy status.

TGF-β/Smad Pathway

The function of transforming growth factor-beta (TGF-β) is connected to remodeling and fibrosis. TGF-β signaling can be improved by ROS.

Impact: When this route is activated, there is an increase in collagen synthesis and fibrosis, which stiffens the cardiac tissue and reduces its ability to function.

In conclusion, oxidative stress affects cardiomyocyte function through a variety of mechanisms and involves a number of signaling pathways. It is a significant factor in the onset and progression of cardiac disease. To reduce the consequences of oxidative stress and enhance cardiovascular health, specific medicines that comprehend these molecular mechanisms are necessary.

THE END

www.ingramcontent.com/pod-product-compliance
Lightning Source LLC
Chambersburg PA
CBHW070125230526
45472CB00004B/1431